I0427346

The complete
manual to thriving
with polycystic
ovarian syndrome
overcoming the root
cause of your
syndrome.
Robinette Hart

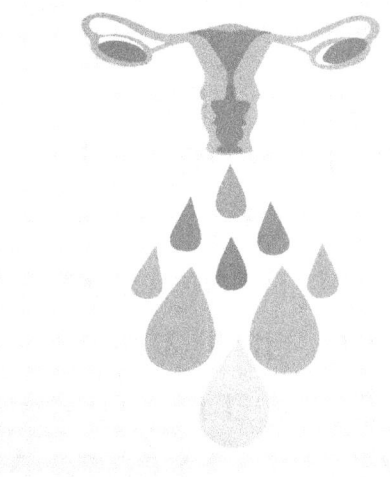

Table of contents.

Introduction

Welcome to the journey of thriving with Polycystic Ovarian Syndrome (PCOS), a comprehensive guide designed to empower and support individuals in overcoming the root causes of this common yet complex health condition. PCOS affects millions of people worldwide, primarily women of reproductive age, and its impact extends beyond the physical realm to influence various aspects of life.

Understanding PCOS:

Polycystic Ovarian Syndrome is characterized by hormonal imbalances, irregular menstrual cycles, and the development of small fluid-filled sacs (cysts) on the ovaries. Beyond its reproductive implications, PCOS can manifest with a range of symptoms, including weight gain, insulin resistance, acne, and hair thinning. The root causes of PCOS are multifaceted, involving genetic, hormonal, and lifestyle factors.

Thriving with PCOS:

This manual is not just about managing symptoms; it's about thriving despite the challenges posed by PCOS. We believe in a holistic approach that goes beyond conventional treatments, focusing on lifestyle modifications, nutrition, and emotional well-being. Thriving with PCOS is not only attainable but can lead to a fulfilling life with improved overall health.

Overcoming Root Causes:

Understanding the root causes of PCOS is crucial for effective management. Hormonal imbalances, insulin resistance, and inflammation are key factors. This manual delves into evidence-based strategies to address these root causes, providing practical insights, dietary recommendations, and lifestyle adjustments to regain hormonal balance and improve overall health.

What to Expect:

Throughout this manual, you will find:

1. Educational Insights:Understand the science behind PCOS, demystifying complex medical concepts in accessible language.
2. Practical Strategies:Implementable tips and strategies to navigate the challenges posed by PCOS in daily life.
3. Nutritional Guidance: Explore a balanced and PCOS-friendly diet that supports hormone regulation and overall well-being.

Chapter one

Welcome

Dear Reader,

Welcome to Thriving with Polycystic Ovarian Syndrome, a guide crafted with care to support you on your journey towards holistic well-being. Whether you've recently been diagnosed or have been living with PCOS for some time, this manual is designed to be your companion, providing valuable insights, practical tips, and a sense of empowerment. Living with PCOS can present challenges, but it is our belief that with the right knowledge and support, you can not only manage the symptoms but also thrive in all aspects of your life. This manual goes beyond the clinical aspects of PCOS, embracing a holistic approach that encompasses your physical, emotional, and mental well-being.

As you navigate these pages, you'll discover a wealth of information, from understanding the science behind PCOS to practical strategies for incorporating positive lifestyle changes. Our goal is to equip you with the tools needed to overcome the root causes of PCOS and embrace a life filled with vitality and resilience. Remember, you're not alone on this journey. We're here to provide guidance, encouragement, and a source of reliable information. Your well-being is our priority, and we hope this manual becomes a source of inspiration as you embark on a path towards thriving with Polycystic Ovarian Syndrome.

Wishing you health, happiness, and empowerment.

Chapter two

What is PCOS and how did I get it

Polycystic Ovarian Syndrome (PCOS) is a common hormonal disorder that affects individuals, primarily women of reproductive age. It is characterized by a combination of symptoms, which can vary in severity and manifestation. PCOS is not fully understood, and its exact cause remains complex, likely involving a combination of genetic, hormonal, and environmental factors.Key Features of PCOS:Irregular Menstrual Cycles: Women with PCOS often experience irregular or absent menstrual periods. This irregularity is a result of hormonal imbalances, particularly elevated levels of androgens, which are male hormones present in both men and women.Ovulatory Dysfunction: PCOS can lead to anovulation, where the ovaries do not release eggs regularly. This can contribute to fertility issues and difficulties in conceiving.Ovarian Cysts:

The condition is named for the presence of small fluid-filled sacs, or cysts, on the ovaries. These cysts are not harmful but can contribute hormonal imbalances.Hyperandrogenism: Elevated levels of androgens, such as testosterone, can lead to physical symptoms like acne, hirsutism (excessive hair growth), and male-pattern baldness.Insulin Resistance: Many individuals with PCOS also exhibit insulin resistance, a condition where the body's cells do not respond effectively to insulin. This can lead to increased insulin levels, contributing to metabolic disturbances.Possible Causes of PCOS:While the exact cause of PCOS is not definitively known, several factors are thought to contribute:Genetics: There appears to be a genetic component, as PCOS often runs in families.Hormonal Imbalances: Elevated levels of androgens, insulin, and luteinizing hormone (LH), along with decreased levels of follicle-stimulating hormone (FSH), contribute to the hormonal disruptions seen in PCOS.Insulin Resistance: Insulin resistance is prevalent in many individuals with

PCOS, leading to increased insulin levels and contributing to the hormonal imbalances.Inflammation: Chronic low-grade inflammation may play a role in the development and progression of PCOS.

Chapter Three

The four step PCOS Repair Protocol to reverse the root cause of your PCOS

Step one: block Androgen for quick Symptom Relief

Androgen blockade plays a crucial role in managing symptoms associated with Polycystic Ovary Syndrome (PCOS). PCOS is characterized by hormonal imbalances, including elevated levels of androgens, such as testosterone. Androgen blockage aims to reduce the effects of these male sex hormones and alleviate symptoms. Here are comprehensive insights into androgen blockade for the relief of PCOS symptoms:
1. Anti-Androgen Medications:Spironolactone:This medication is commonly used to treat hirsutism, acne, and alopecia in women with PCOS. Spironolactone works by blocking androgen receptors,

reducing the impact of androgens on target tissues.

Cyproterone Acetate:* Another anti-androgen, cyproterone acetate, is used to manage hirsutism and regulate menstrual cycles in women with PCOS.

2. Combined Oral Contraceptives:

Birth control pills containing estrogen and progestin are often prescribed to regulate menstrual cycles and reduce androgen levels. These contraceptives can help manage symptoms like irregular periods, acne, and hirsutism.

3. Gonadotropin-Releasing Hormone (GnRH)

Agonists:

Medications like Lupron can be used to suppress ovarian androgen production. GnRH agonists work by temporarily reducing the secretion of gonadotropins, which, in turn, lowers androgen levels.

4. Insulin-Sensitizing Medications:

Insulin resistance is common in PCOS, contributing to elevated androgen levels. Insulin-sensitizing medications like metformin may indirectly lower androgen levels by improving insulin sensitivity.

5. Diet and Lifestyle Modifications

Low-Glycemic Diet:Consuming foods with a low glycemic index helps regulate blood sugar levels, reducing insulin resistance and, consequently, androgen levels.

- Regular Exercise:Physical activity aids in weight management and improves insulin sensitivity, contributing to the reduction of androgen levels.

6. Weight Management:

Losing excess weight can lead to a decrease in androgen levels, as adipose tissue can contribute to hormonal imbalances. A combination of a healthy diet and regular exercise is often recommended.

7. Comprehensive Hormonal Evaluation:

Before initiating androgen blockade, a healthcare professional may conduct thorough hormonal assessments, including levels of testosterone, DHEA-S, and other androgens. This helps tailor treatment to individual needs.

8. Monitoring and Adjustments:

Regular follow-up appointments and hormonal assessments are crucial to monitor the effectiveness of androgen blockade. Adjustments to medication dosages or treatment plans may be made based on individual responses.

9. Potential Side Effects and Considerations:

It's important to be aware of potential side effects of anti-androgen medications, including electrolyte imbalances with spironolactone and menstrual irregularities with GnRH agonists.

Women of childbearing age should use effective contraception, as some medications may pose risks during pregnancy.

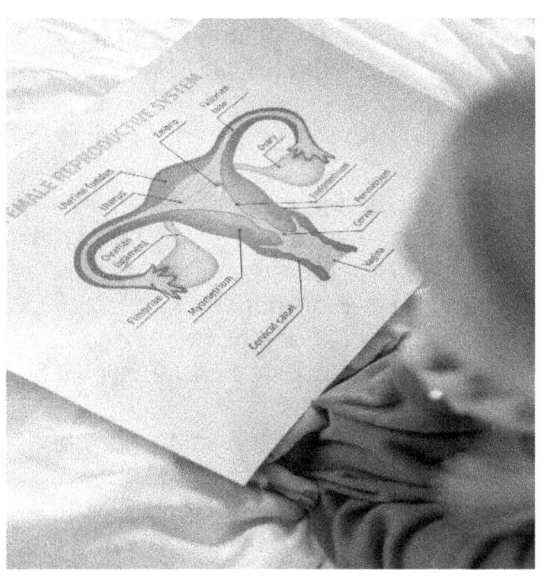

Chapter four
The Anti Androgen plan

The Anti-Androgen Plan is a medical approach aimed at reducing or blocking the effects of androgens, which are male sex hormones, particularly testosterone. This plan is commonly employed in the treatment of conditions such as hirsutism, acne, and transgender hormone therapy.

1. Medications:

   Spironolactone:Often prescribed as an anti-androgen, spironolactone inhibits androgen receptors and reduces testosterone production. It is commonly used for conditions like hirsutism and acne in women.

   Cyproterone Acetate:Another anti-androgen, cyproterone acetate, is used to treat conditions like polycystic ovary syndrome (PCOS) and hirsutism.

2. Hormone Replacement Therapy (HRT):

For Transgender Individuals:Anti-androgen medications may be part of hormone replacement therapy for transgender individuals. Medications like spironolactone or GnRH agonists help suppress testosterone, allowing for feminization.

3. Gonadotropin-Releasing Hormone (GnRH) Agonists:

Lupron and Similar Drugs:These medications work by suppressing the production of gonadotropins, hormones that stimulate the gonads (testes or ovaries). This indirectly leads to a reduction in testosterone levels.

4. Dietary and Lifestyle Changes:

Nutritional Choices: Some foods, like soy products, may have mild anti-androgenic effects. Incorporating a diet rich in fruits, vegetables, and whole grains can contribute to overall hormonal balance.

Exercise: Regular physical activity can help regulate hormone levels, including androgens. It is an important aspect of managing conditions related to androgen excess.

5. Topical Treatments:

Anti-Androgen Creams: Some topical medications containing anti-androgenic agents can be applied directly to the skin. These are often used for conditions like acne or excessive facial hair growth.

6. Monitoring and Adjustments:

Regular Blood Tests:Monitoring hormone levels through blood tests is crucial in adjusting the anti-androgen plan. This ensures that the medication dosage is appropriate and effective.

7. Potential Side Effects:

Bone Health: Prolonged use of some anti-androgens, especially in higher doses, may have an impact on bone health. Regular check-ups and supplements like calcium and vitamin D may be recommended.

It's important to note that any Anti-Androgen Plan should be prescribed and monitored by a qualified healthcare professional, as the effectiveness and potential side effects can vary based on individual health conditions. Regular follow-ups are essential to assess the response to treatment and make necessary adjustments.

Chapter five

The PCOS Repair Breakfast Principal

1.Balanced Macronutrients:A PCOS-friendly breakfast typically includes a balance of macronutrients: carbohydrates, proteins, and healthy fats. This balance helps regulate blood sugar levels and insulin resistance, which are often associated with PCOS.

2. Low Glycemic Index (GI) Carbohydrates:Choose carbohydrates

10. Personalization:Dietary needs can vary among individuals. Some may benefit from a lower-carb approach, while others may find success with different macronutrient ratios. Consulting with a healthcare professional or a registered dietitian for personalized advice is crucial.

Chapter six

PCOS Superfoods

1. Leafy Greens:
   - Rich in antioxidants, leafy greens like spinach and kale can help combat inflammation associated with PCOS.
   High in fiber, aiding in blood sugar regulation and supporting digestive health
2. Berries:
   Blueberries, strawberries, and raspberries are packed with antioxidants, reducing oxidative stress linked to PCOS.
   Low in calories and high in fiber, aiding weight management.
3. Fatty Fish:
   Salmon, mackerel, and sardines contain omega-3 fatty acids, which help reduce inflammation and improve insulin sensitivity.
   Omega-3s also support heart health, crucial for individuals with PCOS who may have a higher risk of cardiovascular issues.
4. Turmeric:

Curcumin, the active compound in turmeric, possesses anti-inflammatory properties.

May aid in managing insulin resistance and hormonal imbalances associated with PCOS.

5. Cinnamon:

Helps regulate insulin levels and may improve insulin sensitivity.

Adds flavor without the need for excessive sugar, promoting better blood sugar control.

6. Nuts and Seeds:

Almonds, walnuts, chia seeds, and flax seeds provide healthy fats, fiber, and essential nutrients.

Supportive weight management and may help balance hormones.

7. Quinoa:

A nutrient-dense, gluten-free grain with a low glycemic index, promoting steady blood sugar levels.

Rich in protein and fiber, aiding in satiety and weight management

8. Greek Yogurt:

High in protein, which can help control appetite and support muscle health.

Probiotics in yogurt contribute to gut health, influencing overall well-being.

9. Avocado:

Provides monounsaturated fats, supporting hormone production and balance.

A nutrient-dense option for managing weight and promoting satiety.

10. Green Tea:

Contains antioxidants known as catechins, which may help manage insulin levels.

Can contribute to weight management and overall metabolic health.

Step Two . Identify your root cause

Identifying the root cause of Polycystic Ovary Syndrome (PCOS) involves understanding the complex interplay of genetic, hormonal, and environmental factors. While the exact cause remains unclear, several contributing factors have been identified:

1. Genetic Predisposition:
   There is a strong genetic component to PCOS, with a higher likelihood of developing the condition if close family members have it.
   Certain gene variants related to insulin signaling, hormone regulation, and inflammation are being investigated for their role in PCOS development.

2. Insulin Resistance:
   Insulin resistance is a key factor in PCOS, where the body's cells become less responsive to insulin, leading to increased insulin levels.
   Elevated insulin levels stimulate the ovaries to produce more androgens (male hormones), contributing to hormonal imbalances.

3. Hormonal Imbalances:
   Elevated levels of androgens, particularly testosterone, are common in individuals with PCOS.
   Disruptions in the balance between luteinizing hormone (LH) and follicle-stimulating hormone (FSH) contribute

to irregular ovulation and the formation of ovarian cysts.

4. Hyperandrogenism:

   Excessive production of androgens by the ovaries and adrenal glands is a hallmark of PCOS.

   This hormonal imbalance can lead to symptoms like hirsutism (excess hair growth), acne, and male-pattern baldness.

5. Inflammation:

   - Chronic low-grade inflammation may play a role in the development and progression of PCOS.

   Inflammatory markers are often elevated in individuals with PCOS, contributing to insulin resistance and other metabolic disturbances.

6. Environmental Factors:

   Exposure to certain environmental factors, such as endocrine-disrupting chemicals (EDCs), may contribute to hormonal imbalances associated with PCOS.

   Lifestyle factors, including diet, physical activity, and stress, can influence PCOS development and symptom severity.

7. Obesity:

   There is a bidirectional relationship between obesity and PCOS, as excess body fat can contribute to insulin resistance and exacerbate hormonal imbalances.

   PCOS itself may also contribute to weight gain, creating a cycle that further worsens symptoms.

8. Gut Microbiota:

   Emerging research suggests a potential link between gut health and PCOS.

Alterations in the gut microbiota may influence inflammation, insulin sensitivity, and hormonal balance. Diagnosing the root cause of PCOS often involves a comprehensive evaluation by healthcare professionals, including a detailed medical history, physical examination, hormonal assessments, and sometimes imaging studies like ultrasound. The multifactorial nature of PCOS requires a personalized approach to management, addressing specific factors contributing to an individual's condition. Lifestyle modifications, such as dietary changes, exercise, and stress management, play a crucial role in managing PCOS and addressing its underlying causes.

Chapter Seven

insulin resistant PCOS (type1)

Insulin-resistant PCOS is a subtype of Polycystic Ovary Syndrome (PCOS) characterized by an impaired response of the body's cells to insulin. Insulin is a hormone produced by the pancreas that plays a crucial role in regulating blood sugar levels and facilitating the uptake of glucose by cells for energy. In individuals with insulin-resistant PCOS, the cells become less responsive to the effects of insulin, leading to a cascade of hormonal and metabolic imbalances.

Mechanisms of Insulin Resistance in PCOS:

1. Hyperinsulinemia:

In response to insulin resistance, the pancreas produces more insulin to compensate for the decreased effectiveness.

Elevated insulin levels stimulate the ovaries to produce excess androgens (male hormones), contributing to the characteristic hormonal imbalances in PCOS.

2. Increased Androgen Production:

Insulin resistance directly influences the ovaries to produce more androgens, particularly testosterone.

Elevated androgen levels contribute to symptoms such as hirsutism, acne, and irregular menstrual cycles.

3. Disruption of Ovulatory Function:
Insulin resistance can disrupt the normal balance between luteinizing hormone (LH) and follicle-stimulating hormone (FSH), leading to irregular ovulation.

Anovulation (lack of ovulation) is a common feature in insulin-resistant PCOS, contributing to infertility.

.4 Weight Gain and Obesity: Insulin resistance is often associated with weight gain and obesity. Excess adipose tissue further exacerbates insulin resistance, creating a cycle that contributes to the severity of PCOS symptoms.

Illustration of Insulin-Resistant PCOS:

1. Initial Insulin Resistance:Cells, particularly in muscles, liver, and adipose tissue, exhibit decreased responsiveness to insulin.

2. Hyperinsulinemia:The pancreas responds by producing more insulin to maintain normal blood sugar levels.

3.Ovarian Response: Elevated insulin levels stimulate the ovaries to produce excess androgens.

4. Hormonal Imbalances: Increased androgens contribute to hirsutism, acne, and interfere with the normal menstrual cycle.

5. Weight Gain and Obesity: Insulin resistance often leads to weight gain, especially in the abdominal region.

Increased adiposity exacerbates insulin resistance, creating a feedback loop.

6. Complications:

Insulin resistance in PCOS is associated with an increased risk of metabolic complications, including type 2 diabetes and cardiovascular disease.

Management of Insulin-Resistant PCOS:

1. Lifestyle Modifications:Regular physical activity helps improve insulin sensitivity and aids in weight management.

Balanced, low-glycemic-index diet to regulate blood sugar levels.

2. Medications: Insulin-sensitizing medications, such as metformin, may be prescribed to improve insulin sensitivity and regulate menstrual cycles.

3. Weight Loss:Achieving and maintaining a healthy weight can significantly improve insulin resistance and reduce symptoms.

4. Hormonal Therapy: Oral contraceptives or anti-androgen medications may be used to regulate

menstrual cycles and manage symptoms related to androgen excess.

Understanding and addressing insulin resistance is crucial in managing PCOS effectively. Tailored interventions that focus on improving insulin sensitivity through lifestyle changes and, if necessary, medications can help mitigate the impact of insulin resistance on the hormonal and metabolic aspects of PCOS.

Chapter eight

Adrenal PCOS (type2)

Adrenal PCOS, also known as adrenal androgen excess, is a subtype of Polycystic Ovary Syndrome (PCOS) characterized by elevated levels of androgens (male hormones) produced by the adrenal glands. While the ovaries are a primary source of androgens in PCOS, in adrenal PCOS, the adrenal glands—situated on top of the kidneys—also contribute significantly to androgen production.

Key Features of Adrenal PCOS

1. Androgen Excess:

Elevated levels of androgens, such as DHEA (dehydroepiandrosterone) and androstenedione, are commonly observed in adrenal PCOS.

Androgen excess contributes to symptoms like hirsutism (excess hair growth), acne, and male-pattern baldness.

2. Irregular Menstrual Cycles:

   Adrenal androgens can disrupt the normal regulation of the menstrual cycle, leading to irregular periods.

   Anovulation (lack of ovulation) is a common consequence, impacting fertility.

3. Cortisol Imbalance:

   Cortisol, another hormone produced by the adrenal glands, may also be affected in adrenal PCOS.

   Chronic stress and elevated cortisol levels can exacerbate hormonal imbalances and contribute to insulin resistance.

4. Insulin Sensitivity:

   Adrenal PCOS may be associated with insulin resistance, influencing the body's ability to regulate blood sugar levels.

   Insulin resistance contributes to metabolic disturbances commonly observed in PCOS.

Causes and Mechanisms:

1. Genetic Factors:

   Genetic predisposition plays a role in the development of adrenal PCOS.

   Variations in genes related to adrenal function and androgen synthesis may contribute.

2. Adrenal Hyperplasia:

   Enlargement or hyperactivity of the adrenal glands may lead to increased androgen production.

   This hyperplasia can be influenced by genetic factors and environmental triggers.

3. Stress and Cortisol:

Chronic stress can stimulate the adrenal glands to produce cortisol, potentially impacting androgen levels.

Elevated cortisol levels may contribute to insulin resistance and hormonal disruptions.

Diagnosis and Evaluation:

1. Hormonal Testing:
   Blood tests measure levels of androgens, including DHEA-S and androstenedione.

   Elevated levels may indicate adrenal androgen excess.
2. Imaging:
   Adrenal imaging, such as an adrenal CT scan or MRI, may be performed to assess the size and function of the adrenal glands.
3. Clinical Evaluation:
   A thorough medical history and physical examination, including an assessment of symptoms, menstrual history, and signs of androgen excess.

Management of Adrenal PCOS:

1. Lifestyle Modifications:
   Stress management techniques, including meditation and relaxation exercises, may help regulate cortisol levels.

   Regular exercise and a balanced diet contribute to overall well-being.
2. Medications:
   Anti-androgen medications, such as spironolactone, may be prescribed to manage symptoms like hirsutism and acne.

Oral contraceptives can regulate menstrual cycles and control androgen excess.

3. Insulin-Sensitizing Agents:
Medications like metformin may be considered to improve insulin sensitivity and address metabolic aspects of PCOS.

4. Addressing Underlying Causes:
Treatment may involve addressing any underlying causes, such as adrenal hyperplasia, through a targeted approach.

Individualized care is essential in managing adrenal PCOS. A healthcare professional will tailor the treatment plan based on the specific hormonal and metabolic imbalances present, as well as addressing any contributing factors such as stress or genetic predisposition. Regular monitoring and collaboration with healthcare providers are crucial for effective management.

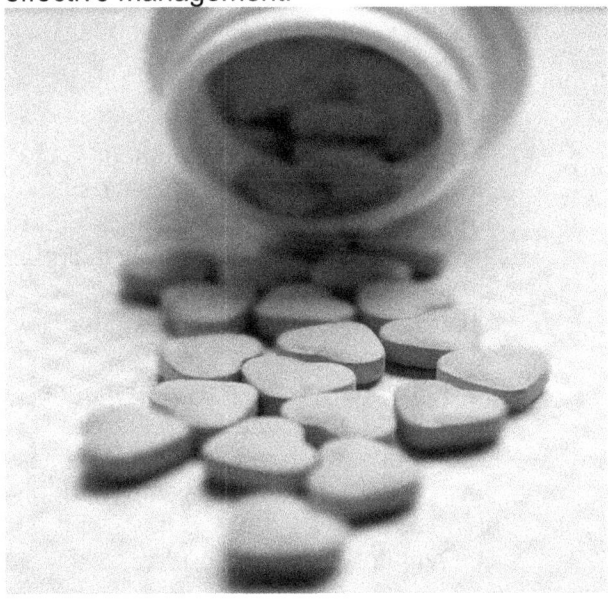

Chapter Nine

Post pill PCOS (type3)

Post-pill PCOS, also known as post-oral contraceptive pill syndrome, refers to a condition where individuals experience symptoms characteristic of Polycystic Ovary Syndrome (PCOS) after discontinuing the use of hormonal contraceptives, such as birth control pills. It's important to note that post-pill PCOS is not officially recognized as a medical diagnosis, but many women report changes in their menstrual cycles and hormonal balance after stopping contraceptive pills.

Key Features of Post-Pill PCOS:

1. Irregular Menstrual Cycles:
   One of the common complaints after discontinuing oral contraceptives is irregular periods.
   Menstrual irregularities may include prolonged cycles, absent periods, or changes in flow.
2. Androgenic Symptoms:
   Some individuals may experience symptoms associated with elevated androgens, such as hirsutism (excess hair growth), acne, and scalp hair thinning.
3. Ovulatory Dysfunction:

Disruption in normal ovulatory function may occur, leading to anovulation (lack of ovulation) and potential fertility challenges.

Causes and Mechanisms:

1. Hormonal Withdrawal:
   Birth control pills suppress natural hormone production, and discontinuation leads to a withdrawal of these synthetic hormones.
   The body may take time to readjust its hormonal balance, and some individuals may experience temporary hormonal imbalances.
2. Rebound Androgen Production:
   Birth control pills often suppress androgen production. After discontinuation, there may be a temporary rebound effect with increased androgen levels.
3. Ovulatory Recovery:
   Some women may experience a delay in the resumption of regular ovulatory cycles after stopping birth control.
   It may take time for the body to regain its natural ovulatory pattern.

Diagnosis and Evaluation:

1. Clinical Presentation:
   Diagnosis is often based on the presentation of symptoms, including irregular menstrual cycles and signs of androgen excess.
2. Hormonal Testing:
   Blood tests may be conducted to assess hormone levels, including androgens and markers of ovarian function.

3. Pelvic Ultrasound:

An ultrasound examination may be performed to evaluate ovarian morphology and the presence of cysts.

Management of Post-Pill PCOS:

1. Observation and Time:

In many cases, the symptoms of post-pill PCOS are temporary, and the body may readjust its hormonal balance over time.

Observation and patience are often recommended, especially if symptoms are not severe.

2. Lifestyle Modifications:

Adopting a healthy lifestyle with regular exercise and a balanced diet can support overall hormonal balance and menstrual regularity.

3. Fertility Awareness:

Individuals trying to conceive should monitor their menstrual cycles and consider fertility awareness methods to identify ovulatory patterns.

4. Medical Intervention:

In cases where symptoms persist or are severe, medical intervention may involve hormonal therapies to regulate menstrual cycles and address androgen excess.

Chapter ten

Inflammatory PCOS (type4)

Inflammatory PCOS refers to a subtype of Polycystic Ovary Syndrome (PCOS) in which chronic inflammation plays a significant role in the development and progression of the condition. Inflammation is a complex immune response that, when chronic, can contribute to hormonal imbalances, insulin resistance, and other metabolic disturbances associated with PCOS.

Key Features of Inflammatory PCOS:

1. Elevated Inflammatory Markers:

Individuals with inflammatory PCOS often exhibit elevated levels of inflammatory markers, such as C-reactive protein (CRP) and pro-inflammatory cytokines.

Chronic inflammation may contribute to the manifestation of PCOS symptoms.

2. Insulin Resistance:

Inflammation can impair insulin signaling pathways, leading to insulin resistance.

Insulin resistance is a common feature of PCOS and can exacerbate hormonal imbalances and contribute to metabolic dysfunction.

3. Ovarian Dysfunction:

Chronic inflammation may disrupt normal ovarian function, leading to irregular ovulation and the formation of ovarian cysts.

- Inflammation can contribute to the elevated production of androgens (male hormones) by the ovaries.

4. Obesity:

Inflammatory PCOS is often associated with obesity, and adipose tissue itself can produce inflammatory substances.

Adipose tissue inflammation contributes to insulin resistance and exacerbates systemic inflammation.

Causes and Mechanisms:

1. Adipose Tissue Inflammation:

Excess adipose tissue, particularly visceral fat, produces inflammatory cytokines.

Adipose tissue inflammation can contribute to insulin resistance and disrupt hormonal balance.

2. Immune System Dysregulation:

Abnormalities in the immune system may contribute to chronic inflammation in PCOS.

Immune cells may infiltrate the ovaries and contribute to the inflammatory environment.

3. Gut Microbiota:

Imbalances in the gut microbiota have been linked to inflammation and insulin resistance in PCOS.

Dysbiosis in the gut may contribute to systemic inflammation.

4. Environmental Factors:

Exposure to environmental pollutants and endocrine-disrupting chemicals (EDCs) may trigger inflammatory responses.

These factors can influence hormonal balance and contribute to PCOS symptoms.

Diagnosis and Evaluation:

1. Inflammatory Markers:

Blood tests measuring inflammatory markers, such as CRP and cytokines, can indicate the presence of inflammation.

2. Clinical Presentation:

Symptoms such as irregular periods, hirsutism, and signs of androgen excess may be present.

3. Pelvic Ultrasound:

An ultrasound may reveal ovarian cysts and provide information about the ovarian morphology.

Management of Inflammatory PCOS:

1. Lifestyle Modifications:

Adopting an anti-inflammatory diet rich in fruits, vegetables, and omega-3 fatty acids can help reduce inflammation.

Regular exercise supports overall health and can have anti-inflammatory effects.

2. Weight Management:

Achieving and maintaining a healthy weight is crucial in managing inflammatory PCOS, as excess adipose tissue contributes to inflammation.

3. Anti-Inflammatory Medications:

Nonsteroidal anti-inflammatory drugs (NSAIDs) may be prescribed to reduce inflammation, but their long-term use requires careful consideration.

4. Treatment of Underlying Causes:

Addressing underlying factors such as gut dysbiosis or environmental exposures may be beneficial.

5. Stress Management:

Chronic stress can contribute to inflammation; therefore, stress management techniques like meditation and yoga may be helpful.

6. Medical Intervention:

In severe cases, healthcare providers may consider medications to manage specific symptoms or underlying inflammation. Managing inflammatory PCOS requires a comprehensive approach addressing both hormonal imbalances and the inflammatory component. Individualized care, considering the unique factors contributing to inflammation in each case, is crucial for effective management. Regular monitoring and collaboration with healthcare providers help tailor interventions for long-term health and symptom control.

Chapter Eleven

The PCOS plate method

The PCOS (Polycystic Ovary Syndrome) plate method is a dietary approach designed to help individuals with PCOS make healthy food choices to manage their symptoms effectively. It focuses on creating balanced meals that support blood sugar control, reduce insulin resistance, and promote overall well-being. The PCOS plate method is a visual guide that divides a plate into specific portions for different food groups.

Components of the PCOS Plate Method:

1. Vegetables (50% of the Plate):
   Fill half of your plate with non-starchy vegetables such as leafy greens, broccoli, cauliflower, peppers, and zucchini.
   Vegetables are rich in fiber, vitamins, and minerals, helping to promote satiety and stabilize blood sugar levels.
2. Protein (25% of the Plate):
   Allocate a quarter of your plate to lean protein sources like poultry, fish, tofu, legumes, or lean meats.
   Protein helps in managing hunger, supporting muscle health, and regulating insulin levels.
3. Whole Grains or Starchy Vegetables (25% of the Plate)
   The remaining quarter of the plate is dedicated to whole grains or starchy vegetables such as quinoa, brown rice, sweet potatoes, or whole-grain pasta.
   Opt for complex carbohydrates with a low glycemic index to promote sustained energy and better blood sugar control.
4. Healthy Fats:
   Incorporate healthy fats in moderation, such as avocados, nuts, seeds, and olive oil.
   Healthy fats contribute to hormone regulation and help in maintaining satiety.
5. Portion Control:
   Pay attention to portion sizes to avoid overeating and support weight management.
   Consistent portion control is essential for regulating calorie intake and insulin sensitivity.

Benefits of the PCOS Plate Method:

1. Blood Sugar Control:
   Balancing the plate with a combination of protein, fiber-rich vegetables, and complex carbohydrates helps regulate blood sugar levels.
   This is particularly important for individuals with PCOS, as insulin resistance is a common feature.
2. Hormonal Balance:
   Including a variety of nutrient-dense foods supports hormonal balance, addressing some of the hormonal imbalances associated with PCOS.
3. Weight Management:
   The PCOS plate method encourages a balanced and nutrient-dense diet, contributing to weight management.
   Maintaining a healthy weight is crucial for managing PCOS symptoms.
4. Satiety and Reduced Cravings:
   The combination of fiber from vegetables and protein helps promote feelings of fullness and reduces cravings for high-calorie, sugary foods.
5. Improved Energy Levels:
   Balanced meals provide sustained energy, reducing energy spikes and crashes often associated with imbalanced diets.
Implementation Tips:
1. Meal Planning:
   Plan meals in advance to ensure a balanced distribution of nutrients.

Include a variety of colorful vegetables and rotate protein sources.
2. Snack Choices:
Apply the PCOS plate method to snacks by incorporating a balance of protein, healthy fats, and whole foods.
3. Hydration:
-Stay hydrated with water or herbal teas to support overall health and well-being.

Chapter twelve

Insulin resistant core treat

Insulin resistance is a condition where the body's cells become less responsive to the effects of insulin, a hormone that helps regulate blood sugar. Managing insulin resistance is crucial to preventing complications such as type 2 diabetes and cardiovascular issues. Here's an overview of core treatments:
1. Lifestyle Modifications:
Diet: Focus on a balanced, low-glycemic diet with emphasis on whole grains, lean proteins, healthy fats, and plenty of vegetables.
Exercise: Regular physical activity improves insulin sensitivity. Both aerobic and resistance training are beneficial.
2. Weight Management:
Achieving and maintaining a healthy weight is pivotal in improving insulin sensitivity.

Weight loss through a combination of diet and exercise is often recommended.

3. Medications:

Metformin: Commonly prescribed to manage insulin resistance, it helps lower blood sugar levels and improves insulin sensitivity.

Thiazolidinediones (TZDs): These medications enhance insulin sensitivity in the muscles and fat tissues.

Incretin-based therapies:Drugs like GLP-1 agonists and DPP-4 inhibitors help regulate blood sugar and may improve insulin sensitivity.

4. Insulin Sensitizers:

Certain supplements and herbs, like berberine and cinnamon, may have insulin-sensitizing properties. However, their efficacy varies, and it's essential to consult a healthcare professional before incorporating them.

5. Monitor Blood Sugar Levels:

Regular monitoring helps track progress and adjust treatment plans accordingly.

Continuous glucose monitoring (CGM) devices provide real-time data, aiding in better management.

6. Stress Management:

Chronic stress can contribute to insulin resistance. Practices such as mindfulness, meditation, and adequate sleep can help manage stress levels.

7. Smoking Cessation:

Smoking has been linked to insulin resistance. Quitting smoking is beneficial not only for overall health but also in managing insulin resistance.

8. Medical Supervision:
   Regular check-ups with healthcare professionals are essential for monitoring progress, adjusting medications, and addressing any emerging issues.

9. Personalized Approach:
   Treatment plans should be tailored to individual needs, considering factors like age, overall health, and coexisting medical conditions.

It's important to note that managing insulin resistance is a lifelong process, and adherence to a holistic approach, combining lifestyle modifications and medical interventions, is key for successful outcomes. Always consult with a healthcare professional to create a personalized treatment plan based on your specific health status.

Chapter thirteen

Adrenal PCOS core treatment

Adrenal PCOS, also known as adrenal androgen excess or adrenal-related polycystic ovary syndrome, is a subtype of PCOS (Polycystic Ovary Syndrome) where elevated levels of adrenal androgens play a significant role in the condition. Treatment for adrenal PCOS often involves addressing the underlying hormonal imbalances and managing symptoms. Here's a detailed overview of the core treatment:

1. Hormonal Regulation:

Anti-androgen Medications: Drugs such as spironolactone or flutamide may be prescribed to reduce androgen levels and alleviate symptoms like hirsutism (excessive hair growth) and acne.

Oral Contraceptives (OCs): Birth control pills can help regulate menstrual cycles and reduce androgen levels by suppressing the ovaries' production of androgens.

2. Glucocorticoid Therapy:

For cases where elevated adrenal androgens are prominent, low-dose glucocorticoids like dexamethasone or prednisone may be prescribed to suppress adrenal androgen production.

3. Lifestyle Modifications:

Weight Management: Achieving and maintaining a healthy weight is crucial in managing adrenal PCOS.

Dietary Changes: Adopting a low-glycemic diet with a focus on whole foods, lean proteins, and complex carbohydrates can help regulate insulin levels, which in turn may positively impact androgen levels.

4. Exercise:

Regular physical activity has been shown to improve insulin sensitivity and regulate hormonal imbalances, including those related to PCOS.

5. Nutritional Supplements:

Inositol: Particularly myo-inositol and D-chiro-inositol have shown promise in improving insulin sensitivity and ovarian function in women with PCOS.

Vitamin D: Adequate levels of vitamin D are important for hormonal balance, and supplementation may be recommended if levels are deficient.

6. Addressing Insulin Resistance:

Medications such as metformin, commonly used in PCOS treatment, may be prescribed to improve insulin sensitivity.

7. Regular Monitoring:

Periodic evaluations of hormonal levels, lipid profiles, and glucose metabolism are important to assess the effectiveness of treatment and make adjustments as needed.

8. Fertility Management:

For women with fertility concerns, ovulation-inducing medications like letrozole or clomiphene citrate may be considered under medical supervision.

9. Psychological Support:

PCOS can have a significant impact on mental health. Counseling or support groups may be beneficial in addressing psychological aspects and improving overall well-being.

10. Individualized Approach:

Treatment plans should be tailored to the individual, considering factors such as age, reproductive goals, and co-existing health conditions. Adrenal PCOS management often requires a multidisciplinary approach involving endocrinologists, gynecologists, nutritionists, and possibly mental health professionals. It's crucial to consult with healthcare providers to develop a personalized treatment plan based on a thorough assessment of the individual's specific health status and needs.

Chapter fourteen

Post pill PCOS core treatment

Post-pill PCOS refers to the development of polycystic ovary syndrome (PCOS) symptoms after discontinuing hormonal contraceptives, such as birth control pills. Treatment for post-pill PCOS involves addressing hormonal imbalances, managing symptoms, and promoting overall reproductive health. Here's a detailed overview of the core treatment:

1. Hormonal Evaluation:
   Comprehensive hormonal assessments, including levels of androgens (testosterone), LH (luteinizing hormone), FSH (follicle-stimulating hormone), and estrogen, help identify specific imbalances.

2. Lifestyle Modifications:
   - Dietary Changes: Adopting a low-glycemic diet with emphasis on whole foods, lean proteins, and complex carbohydrates can help regulate insulin levels, which may be disrupted after discontinuing hormonal contraceptives.
   - Weight Management: Achieving and maintaining a healthy weight is crucial, as excess body fat can contribute to hormonal imbalances associated with PCOS.

3. Insulin Sensitivity:
   - Medications like metformin may be prescribed to improve insulin

sensitivity, addressing any insulin resistance that may have developed.

4. Ovulation Induction:
   - For women experiencing irregular or absent menstrual cycles, medications such as letrozole or clomiphene citrate may be used to induce ovulation under medical supervision.

5. Anti-Androgen Medications:
   - Drugs like spironolactone or flutamide may be prescribed to manage symptoms such as hirsutism (excessive hair growth) and acne by reducing androgen levels.

6. Oral Contraceptives (OCs):
   - While discontinuation of birth control pills may have triggered the development of post-pill PCOS, in some cases, restarting OCs may be considered to regulate menstrual cycles and manage symptoms. However, this is typically a temporary solution.

7. Nutritional Supplements:
   - Inositol: Myo-inositol and D-chiro-inositol supplementation has shown promise in improving insulin sensitivity and ovarian function in women with PCOS.
   - Vitamin D: Adequate levels of vitamin D are important for hormonal balance, and supplementation may be recommended if levels are deficient.

8. Fertility Management:
   - Women concerned about fertility may undergo assisted reproductive technologies (ART) under the guidance of a fertility specialist.

9. Monitoring and Follow-Up:
   - Regular monitoring of hormonal levels, menstrual cycles, and overall

health is crucial. Adjustments to the treatment plan can be made based on individual responses and evolving needs.

10. Psychological Support:
   - Coping with PCOS symptoms, especially after discontinuing contraceptives, can be challenging. Counseling or support groups may provide valuable emotional support.

11. Individualized Approach:
   - Treatment plans should be personalized, taking into account factors such as age, reproductive goals, and co-existing health conditions. Close collaboration with healthcare providers is essential for ongoing care and adjustments to the treatment plan.

It's important for individuals with post-pill PCOS to consult with healthcare professionals, including endocrinologists and gynecologists, to develop a comprehensive and tailored treatment approach. This ensures that the management strategy addresses the specific hormonal imbalances and symptoms unique to each individual.

Chapter fifteen

Inflammatory PCOS core treatment

Inflammatory PCOS, sometimes referred to as Inflammatory Polycystic Ovary Syndrome, is a subtype of PCOS where chronic inflammation plays a significant role in the development and progression of the condition. The treatment for inflammatory PCOS involves addressing inflammation, hormonal imbalances, and associated symptoms. Here's a comprehensive overview of the core treatment:

1. Inflammation Management:
   - Anti-Inflammatory Diet:Adopting a diet rich in anti-inflammatory foods, such as fruits, vegetables, whole grains, and omega-3 fatty acids, may help reduce inflammation.
   - Omega-3 Supplements: Fish oil or flaxseed oil supplements, containing omega-3 fatty acids, have anti-inflammatory properties and may be recommended.

2. Hormonal Regulation:
   - Combined Oral Contraceptives (COCs):Birth control pills are often prescribed to regulate menstrual cycles and reduce androgen levels, addressing hormonal imbalances associated with PCOS.
   Anti-Androgen Medications: Drugs like spironolactone may be used to manage symptoms like hirsutism and acne by reducing androgen levels.

3. Insulin Sensitivity:
   Medications such as metformin may be prescribed to improve insulin sensitivity, especially if insulin resistance is contributing to the inflammatory aspects of PCOS.

4. Lifestyle Modifications:
   Regular Exercise: Physical activity has anti-inflammatory effects and helps improve insulin sensitivity. Both aerobic and resistance training can be beneficial.
   Weight Management:Achieving and maintaining a healthy weight is crucial,

as excess body fat can contribute to inflammation and exacerbate PCOS symptoms.

5. Nutritional Supplements:

Inositol: Myo-inositol and D-chiro-inositol supplementation may improve insulin sensitivity and ovarian function, potentially addressing inflammatory aspects of PCOS.

Vitamin D: Adequate levels of vitamin D are important for immune function and may have anti-inflammatory effects.

6. Stress Management:

Chronic stress can contribute to inflammation. Techniques such as mindfulness, meditation, and yoga may be recommended for stress reduction.

7. Anti-Inflammatory Medications:

In some cases, nonsteroidal anti-inflammatory drugs (NSAIDs) may be prescribed to manage pain associated with inflammation.

8. Fertility Management:

Ovulation-inducing medications like letrozole or clomiphene citrate may be considered for women experiencing fertility concerns due to irregular ovulation.

9. Regular Monitoring:

Periodic evaluations of hormonal levels, inflammation markers, and overall health are crucial to assess the effectiveness of treatment and make adjustments as needed.

10. Psychological Support:

Living with a chronic condition can impact mental health. Counseling or support groups may be beneficial for managing the emotional aspects of PCOS.

11. Individualized Approach:
  Treatment plans should be personalized, considering factors such as age, reproductive goals, and co-existing health conditions. Close collaboration with healthcare providers is essential for ongoing care and adjustments to the treatment plan. Addressing inflammatory PCOS involves a holistic approach that considers both lifestyle modifications and medical interventions. Consultation with healthcare professionals, including endocrinologists and gynecologists, is crucial to developing a comprehensive and individualized treatment plan.

Chapter sixteen

Nutrient deficiencies,testing and supplements

Polycystic Ovary Syndrome (PCOS) is a complex endocrine disorder that can be associated with nutrient deficiencies. Proper testing, identification, and supplementation of these deficiencies play a crucial role in the management of PCOS. Here's a comprehensive overview:
Nutrient Deficiencies in PCOS:
1. Vitamin D:
  Deficiency Impact:Linked to insulin resistance and menstrual irregularities.
  Testing: Serum 25-hydroxyvitamin D levels.

Supplementation: Vitamin D supplements if levels are insufficient.

2. Inositol:

Deficiency Impact: Impaired insulin sensitivity and ovarian function.

Testing: Limited direct testing; often assessed through symptoms and risk factors.

Supplementation: Myo-inositol and D-chiro-inositol supplements can be beneficial.

3. Omega-3 Fatty Acids:

Deficiency Impact: Altered lipid profiles and increased inflammation.

Testing: No specific test for omega-3 levels; often assessed through dietary intake and symptoms.

Supplementation: Fish oil or flaxseed oil supplements.

4. B Vitamins (especially B12 and Folate):

Deficiency Impact: Influences insulin resistance and overall metabolic health.

Testing: Serum levels of B12 and folate.

Supplementation: B12 or folate supplements if levels are deficient.

5. Iron:

Deficiency Impact: Anemia, fatigue, and menstrual irregularities.

Testing: Serum ferritin levels.

Supplementation: Iron supplements if deficiency is detected.

Nutrient Testing in PCOS:

1. Blood Tests:

Comprehensive blood tests for hormones, lipids, and metabolic markers can help identify deficiencies and assess overall health.

Hormonal markers include androgens, estrogen, and progesterone.

2. Vitamin D Testing:

Serum 25-hydroxyvitamin D levels are measured to determine vitamin D status.

Optimal levels are generally considered to be 30-50 ng/mL.

3. Inositol Levels:

Direct testing for inositol levels is not widely available.

Assessment is often based on symptoms, medical history, and risk factors.

4. Nutrient Panel:

A comprehensive nutrient panel can evaluate levels of various vitamins and minerals associated with PCOS.

Nutrient Supplementation in PCOS:

1. Vitamin D:

Supplements are common if deficiency is identified. Dosage depends on severity.

2. Inositol:

Supplementation with myo-inositol and D-chiro-inositol in specific ratios can improve insulin sensitivity and ovarian function.

3. Omega-3 Fatty Acids:

Fish oil or flaxseed oil supplements can provide essential omega-3 fatty acids.

4. B Vitamins:

B12 or folate supplements may be recommended if deficiency is detected.

5. Iron:

Iron supplements may be prescribed for those with iron deficiency anemia.

Considerations:

1. Individualized Approach:
   Nutrient needs vary, and supplementation should be tailored to individual deficiencies.
2. Professional Guidance:
   Consultation with a healthcare professional, preferably a nutritionist or dietitian, is essential for personalized advice.
3. Monitoring:
   - Regular monitoring of nutrient levels is important to adjust supplementation as needed.
4. Whole Foods:
   Emphasize a balanced diet with nutrient-dense whole foods as the primary source of nutrients.
5. Caution with Supplements:
   While supplementation is important, excessive intake can have adverse effects. It's crucial to follow recommended dosages.

addressing nutrient deficiencies in PCOS involves comprehensive testing, individualized supplementation, and ongoing monitoring to support overall health and manage specific symptoms associated with the condition. Always seek guidance from healthcare professionals for personalized advice based on your specific health status

Chapter seventeen
Sleep for cysters

Establishing a healthy sleep schedule is crucial for individuals with polycystic ovary syndrome (PCOS), often referred to as cysters. Sleep plays a vital role in hormonal regulation, metabolism, and overall well-being. Here's a comprehensive guide on creating a beneficial sleep schedule for those with PCOS:

Importance of Sleep for PCOS:

1. Hormonal Balance:

Quality sleep supports the regulation of hormones such as insulin, cortisol, and reproductive hormones like estrogen and progesterone.

Hormonal imbalances are common in PCOS, and adequate sleep can help mitigate these issues.

2. Metabolic Health:

Sleep is linked to metabolic processes, and disruptions can contribute to insulin resistance, a common concern in PCOS.

Consistent sleep patterns support better glucose metabolism.

3. Weight Management:

Lack of sleep is associated with weight gain and obesity, which can exacerbate PCOS symptoms.

Adequate sleep supports weight management efforts.

4. Stress Reduction:

Proper sleep helps manage stress levels and reduces cortisol, a stress hormone.

Chronic stress is known to contribute to PCOS symptoms.

5. Mood and Mental Health:

Sleep influences mood and cognitive function.

Poor sleep quality is linked to increased risk of depression and anxiety, which can impact overall well-being in individuals with PCOS.

Creating a Healthy Sleep Schedule for Cysters:

1. Consistent Bedtime:

Aim for a regular bedtime and wake-up time, even on weekends.

Consistency helps regulate the body's internal clock.

2. Bedtime Routine:

Establish a calming routine before bedtime, such as reading, gentle stretching, or meditation.

Avoid stimulating activities and electronic devices close to bedtime.

3. Optimal Sleep Duration:

Adults generally need 7-9 hours of sleep per night.

Find the duration that leaves you feeling refreshed and alert during the day.

4. Sleep Environment:

Create a comfortable sleep environment with a cool, dark, and quiet bedroom.

Invest in a supportive mattress and pillows.

5. Limit Caffeine and Stimulants:

Avoid caffeine and stimulants in the hours leading up to bedtime.

Be mindful of hidden sources of caffeine in medications and certain foods.

6. Regular Exercise:

Engage in regular physical activity, but avoid intense exercise close to bedtime.

Exercise promotes better sleep quality.

7. Balanced Diet:

Maintain a balanced diet with regular meals.

Avoid heavy meals close to bedtime, but a light snack may be helpful if you are hungry.

8. Manage Stress:

Practice stress-reducing techniques such as deep breathing, meditation, or yoga.

Consider journaling to unload thoughts before bedtime.

9. Limit Naps:

If you nap during the day, keep it short (20-30 minutes) and avoid late-afternoon naps.

10. Seek Professional Help:

If sleep difficulties persist, consult a healthcare professional for guidance.

Sleep disorders such as sleep apnea should be addressed.

Monitoring Sleep Patterns:

1. Sleep Diary:

Keep a sleep diary to track bedtime, wake-up time, and sleep quality.

Note any factors affecting sleep, such as stress or dietary changes.

2. Wearable Devices:

Consider using wearable devices or apps to monitor sleep patterns.

These tools can provide insights into sleep duration and quality.

3. Professional Evaluation:

If sleep issues persist, consult with a sleep specialist or healthcare provider for a thorough evaluation. Establishing and maintaining a healthy sleep schedule is a crucial aspect of overall PCOS management. By prioritizing sleep and implementing consistent sleep habits, individuals with PCOS can support hormonal balance, metabolic health, and overall well-being. It's important to address sleep as part of a holistic approach to managing PCOS symptoms.

Chapter Eighteen

Movement and exercise for PCOS

Physical activity and exercise play a significant role in managing Polycystic Ovary Syndrome (PCOS). Regular movement not only helps with weight management but also improves insulin sensitivity, lowers inflammation, and promotes overall well-being. Here's a detailed guide on movement and exercise for individuals with PCOS:

Types of Exercise Beneficial for PCOS:

1. Aerobic Exercise:
   Benefits: Improves cardiovascular health, aids in weight loss, and enhances insulin sensitivity.
   Examples: Brisk walking, jogging, cycling, swimming, and aerobic classes.

2. Resistance Training:
   Benefits: Builds muscle mass, increases metabolism, and enhances insulin sensitivity.
   Examples: Weight lifting, bodyweight exercises, resistance band workouts.

3. High-Intensity Interval Training (HIIT):
   Benefits: Efficient for fat loss, improves insulin sensitivity, and boosts cardiovascular fitness.
   Examples: Short bursts of intense activity followed by brief periods of rest or lower-intensity exercise.

4. Yoga:

Benefits: Reduces stress, improves flexibility, and may help regulate hormonal balance.

Examples: Hatha, Vinyasa, or Restorative yoga.

5. Pilates:

Benefits: Strengthens core muscles, improves flexibility, and enhances overall body strength.

Examples: Mat-based or equipment-based Pilates exercises.

Exercise Guidelines for PCOS:

1. Frequency:

Aim for at least 150 minutes of moderate-intensity aerobic exercise or 75 minutes of vigorous-intensity exercise per week.

Include resistance training at least two days a week.

2. Consistency:

Establish a consistent exercise routine, incorporating both aerobic and resistance training.

Gradually increase intensity and duration as fitness improves.

3. Individualization:

Choose activities you enjoy to increase adherence.

Modify exercises based on fitness level, any existing health conditions, or injuries.

4. Balanced Approach:

Combine aerobic and resistance training for a well-rounded fitness routine.

Include flexibility and balance exercises, such as yoga or Pilates.

5. Gradual Progression:

Start with manageable durations and intensities, especially for beginners.

Progress gradually to avoid overtraining or injury.

6. Mindful Movement:

Focus on mindful movement to reduce stress.

Practices like tai chi or walking in nature can enhance mental well-being.

7. Posture Awareness:

Emphasize proper posture during exercises, especially if sitting for extended periods is common.

Core-strengthening exercises can improve posture.

Tips for Incorporating Exercise into PCOS Management:

1. Consultation with Healthcare Providers:

Before starting a new exercise regimen, consult with healthcare providers, especially if there are existing health concerns.

2. Variety and Fun:

Include a variety of exercises to prevent boredom and maintain interest.

Engage in activities that bring joy to make the routine more sustainable.

3. Supportive Community:

Join exercise classes or groups to build a supportive community.

Social support can enhance motivation.

4. Monitoring Progress:

Track progress to stay motivated.

Monitor changes in weight, fitness levels, and improvements in PCOS symptoms.

5. Adaptability:

Be adaptable to life changes.

Modify the exercise routine as needed during different life stages.

6. Rest and Recovery:
   Prioritize rest and recovery days to prevent burnout.
   Listen to the body and adjust intensity when necessary.
Potential Challenges and Considerations:
1. Hormonal Fluctuations:
   Adapt the exercise routine to accommodate energy levels during different phases of the menstrual cycle.
2. Individual Differences:
   PCOS symptoms vary among individuals.
   Tailor exercise plans based on individual health, preferences, and goals.
3. Professional Guidance:
   Consider working with fitness professionals, such as personal trainers or physical therapists, for personalized guidance and support.
Exercise is a cornerstone in the holistic management of PCOS. A well-designed and consistently followed exercise routine, along with a healthy diet and lifestyle, can contribute significantly to improving metabolic health, hormonal balance, and overall quality of life for individuals with PCOS.

Chapter nineteen

Getting pregnant with PCOS

Getting pregnant with Polycystic Ovary Syndrome (PCOS) can present challenges due to irregular ovulation and hormonal imbalances. However, with proper management and lifestyle adjustments, many individuals with PCOS can successfully conceive. Here's a detailed guide on the steps to enhance fertility and increase the chances of getting pregnant with PCOS:

1. Medical Assessment:

Consult with a Reproductive Endocrinologist or Gynecologist:

Seek professional guidance to assess fertility and determine the best course of action.

- Discuss any underlying conditions, such as insulin resistance, that may impact fertility.

2. Cycle Monitoring and Ovulation Prediction:

Regular Cycle Monitoring:

Track menstrual cycles to identify patterns and assess ovulation.

Utilize fertility awareness methods or ovulation predictor kits.

3. Lifestyle Modifications:

Healthy Diet:

Adopt a balanced and nutritious diet to support overall health and address insulin resistance.

Focus on whole foods, complex carbohydrates, lean proteins, and healthy fats.

Weight Management:

Achieve and maintain a healthy weight.

Weight loss, even a modest amount, can improve ovulation and increase fertility.

Regular Exercise:

Engage in regular physical activity to promote overall well-being.

Moderate exercise can help regulate insulin levels and improve fertility.

Stress Management:
Practice stress-reducing techniques such as mindfulness, meditation, or yoga.

Chronic stress can negatively impact fertility.

Adequate Sleep:
Ensure sufficient and quality sleep to support hormonal balance.

Aim for 7-9 hours of sleep per night.

4. Medical Interventions:
Ovulation-Inducing Medications:
Clomiphene citrate or letrozole may be prescribed to induce ovulation.

These medications stimulate the ovaries to release eggs.

Metformin:
For individuals with insulin resistance, metformin may be recommended to improve hormonal balance and ovulation.

Injectable Gonadotropins:
In more severe cases, injectable medications like FSH may be prescribed to stimulate ovulation.

In Vitro Fertilization (IVF):
IVF may be considered if other treatments are unsuccessful.

Fertilized eggs are implanted into the uterus

Laparoscopic Ovarian Drilling:
A surgical procedure that can be considered to induce ovulation by making small holes in the ovaries.

5. Support from a Fertility Specialist:
Consultation with a Fertility Specialist:

For individuals facing challenges, seeking guidance from a fertility specialist is crucial.

Comprehensive fertility assessments and personalized treatment plans can be developed.

6. Patience and Emotional Well-Being:
   Emotional Support:
   Infertility can be emotionally challenging. Seek support from loved ones, friends, or support groups.

   Consider counseling or therapy if needed.

   Patience and Persistence:
   It may take time to achieve pregnancy.

   Be patient and stay committed to the recommended treatment plan.

7. Monitoring and Adjustments:
   Regular Follow-ups:
   Regularly consult with healthcare providers to monitor progress.

   Adjustments to the treatment plan may be made based on individual responses.

8. Preconception Care:
   Prenatal Vitamins:
   Begin taking prenatal vitamins containing folic acid before conception.

   Ensure the body has essential nutrients for a   healthy pregnancy.

   Optimize Health
   Address any pre-existing health conditions.

   Optimize overall health for a smoother pregnancy.

It's important to note that the journey to pregnancy with PCOS is unique for each individual. Consulting with healthcare professionals, including fertility specialists, can provide personalized guidance and increase the likelihood of a successful pregnancy. Patience, persistence, and a comprehensive approach to health and fertility are key elements in the process.

Chapter twenty

Step :3 find a community of moving forward

Finding a supportive community is crucial for individuals with Polycystic Ovary Syndrome (PCOS). Connecting with others who share similar experiences can provide valuable emotional support, information, and encouragement. Here's a detailed guide on how to find and engage with a community while highlighting its importance for PCOS patients:
How to Find a Community:
1. Online Platforms:
    Social Media Groups:
    Join PCOS-specific groups on platforms like Facebook, Reddit, or Instagram.
    Search for keywords like PCOS support or PCOS community.
    Forums and Websites:
    Explore forums and websites dedicated to PCOS.
    Websites like SoulCysters or PCOS Challenge often provide community forums.
2. Local Support Groups:
    Check Local Healthcare Providers:

Inquire with healthcare providers or clinics specializing in PCOS for information on local support groups.
Meetup Groups:
Use Meetup.com or similar platforms to find local PCOS support groups or wellness events.
3. Health Organizations:
PCOS Advocacy Organizations:
Connect with organizations like PCOS Challenge, which often provide resources and opportunities to engage with the community.
Women's Health Clinics:
Contact women's health clinics or reproductive health centers for information on local support networks.
4. Educational Events:
Attend Workshops or Webinars:
Participate in workshops or webinars on PCOS organized by healthcare providers, advocacy groups, or wellness organizations.
Conferences:
Attend conferences focused on women's health or PCOS.
Many conferences offer opportunities for networking and connecting with others.
Importance of Community for PCOS Patients:
1. Emotional Support:
Shared Experiences:
Connecting with others who understand the challenges of PCOS provides a sense of camaraderie.
Shared experiences can validate one's feelings and reduce feelings of isolation.
Encouragement and Motivation:

A supportive community offers encouragement during both successes and setbacks.

Motivation from others can be instrumental in managing lifestyle changes

2. Information and Resources:
Shared Knowledge:
Communities often share valuable information about PCOS management, treatment options, and lifestyle tips.

Members may provide insights based on their own experiences.
Access to Experts:
Some communities may have access to healthcare professionals, nutritionists, or experts who can answer questions and provide guidance.

3. Holistic Well-Being:
Mental Health:
Connecting with others promotes mental well-being.

Sharing coping strategies and discussing mental health aspects can be therapeutic.
Lifestyle Support:
Communities may offer advice on adopting a healthier lifestyle, including diet and exercise recommendations.

4. Advocacy and Awareness:
Collective Advocacy:
Joining a community allows individuals to contribute to PCOS advocacy efforts.

Collective voices can raise awareness and push for better understanding and research on PCOS.

5. Friendship and Networking:
Building Relationships:

Friendships often form within these communities, providing a network of support.

Networking can lead to opportunities for shared activities or collaboration on wellness goals.

6. Shared Coping Strategies:

Coping Mechanisms:

Communities offer a platform to share effective coping strategies for managing PCOS-related symptoms and challenges.

Peer-to-Peer Support:

Learning from others who have successfully coped with similar issues can be empowering.

Tips for Engaging in a Community:

1. Active Participation:

Contribute and Share:

Actively participate in discussions, share your experiences, and ask questions.

Contribution strengthens the sense of community.

2. Respect and Empathy:

Be Respectful:

Respect diverse opinions and experiences within the community.

Show empathy towards others who may be going through difficult times.

3. Verify Information:

Fact-Checking:

Verify information received within the community, especially related to medical advice.

Consult healthcare professionals for personalized guidance.

4. Set Healthy Boundaries:

Balanced Engagement:

Engage with the community in a way that is beneficial without becoming overwhelming.

Set boundaries to protect your mental well-being.

5. Privacy Considerations:

Mindful Sharing:

Be mindful of the information you share online.

Protect your privacy while still benefiting from the support of the community.

Building and maintaining connections within a PCOS community is a powerful resource for individuals navigating the challenges of this condition. It offers a sense of belonging, access to valuable information, and a platform for shared empowerment and advocacy. Remember that each person's journey with PCOS is unique, and finding a supportive community can contribute significantly to overall well-being and resilience.

Conclusions

In concluding the comprehensive manual to thriving with Polycystic Ovary Syndrome (PCOS), it is evident that navigating this condition requires a multifaceted and personalized approach. From understanding the intricacies of PCOS to implementing lifestyle changes, seeking medical guidance, and fostering a supportive community, individuals with PCOS have the tools to not just manage but thrive in their journey.

Thriving with PCOS involves acknowledging the unique challenges it presents, embracing lifestyle modifications that promote hormonal balance and overall well-being, and seeking support from both healthcare professionals and fellow PCOS warriors. The manual emphasizes the importance of education, self-awareness, and the power of community in overcoming obstacles and celebrating victories, no matter how small.

As we conclude, remember that thriving is not about erasing the challenges but about navigating them with resilience, courage, and a commitment to self-care. By embracing a holistic approach that addresses physical, emotional, and mental aspects, individuals with PCOS can live vibrant, fulfilling lives

In this journey, empowerment comes from knowledge, self-compassion, and the support of a community that understands the complexities of PCOS. Let this manual serve as a guide, a source of inspiration, and a reminder that thriving with PCOS is not only possible but within reach for each person determined to take charge of their health and well-being. May the path to thriving with PCOS be paved with resilience, self-love, and the strength derived from the collective spirit of those who face and conquer the challenge.